Marwa BOUSSAID
Rakia SOINIYA
Abir AISSAOUI

Patient rights

Marwa BOUSSAID
Rakia SOINIYA
Abir AISSAOUI

Patient rights

Assessing healthcare professionals' knowledge of patients' rights

ScienciaScripts

Cover image: www.ingimage.com

This book is a translation from the original published under ISBN 978-620-6-72078-2.

Publisher:
Sciencia Scripts
is a trademark of
Dodo Books Indian Ocean Ltd. and OmniScriptum S.R.L publishing group

120 High Road, East Finchley, London, N2 9ED, United Kingdom
Str. Armeneasca 28/1, office 1, Chisinau MD-2012, Republic of Moldova, Europe
Printed at: see last page
ISBN: 978-620-8-07171-4

TABLE OF CONTENTS

I. CHAPTER 1: INTRODUCTION 3

II. CHAPTER 2: Patients' rights 8

A. Right to life : 8

B. Right to care :... 13

C. The right to personal dignity and integrity :. 15

D. Right to inviolability of the body :................ 17

E. Right to non-discrimination :....................... 20

F. Right to confidentiality : 21

G. Right to information :.................................. 23

H. Consent to care :... 25

I. Right to free choice of caregiver and access to medical records :... 27

J. Right to compensation for any damage :......... 29

III. CHAPTER 3: Assessing the knowledge of medical staff... 32

A. Materials and methods : 32

1. Type of study :.. 32
2. Study population : 32
3. Data collection :.. 33
4. Data analysis :... 35
5. Descriptive section 35

6. Analytical part 36
7. Ethical considerations : 37

B. Results of the medical staff knowledge assessment 37

1. Part 1: Assessment of medical staff's knowledge of health law and ethics 37
2. Part 2: Assessment of medical staff's knowledge of the health rights of persons deprived of their liberty.. 43

C. Discussion of results : 46

1. Factors influencing the level of knowledge : 47
2. Right to information : 49
3. Right to consent : 52
4. Right to choice of doctor and access to medical records : 56
5. Medical confidentiality : 58
6. Drug research :.. 67
7. Non-assistance to a person in danger : 74

IV. CHAPTER 4: Recommendations : 78

V. CHAPTER 5: Conclusions 83

VI. References : 85

VII. Appendices 93

I. CHAPTER 1: INTRODUCTION

Patients' rights are an essential pillar of modern healthcare systems, founded on the fundamental principles of human rights. These rights are inalienable and universal, irrespective of socio-economic, ethnic, gender, age or any other form of discrimination.

Patient rights are based on the recognition of health as an essential element of individual and collective well-being. This principle was first set out in the Constitution of the World Health Organization (WHO) in 1946, which declared that "*the health of all peoples is fundamental to the attainment of the highest possible level of health by each individual*".(1). This affirmation was further reinforced by Article 3 of the Universal Declaration of Human Rights, which enshrines the inherent right of everyone to life, liberty and security of person(2).

These rights, established by deontological and legal standards, proclaim the intangibility of human dignity in the face of illness. Their protection is of crucial importance given the vulnerability of the patient, weakened by illness and dependent on healthcare professionals.

Over the centuries, these rights - rooted in the doctor-patient relationship, often perceived as a moral contract between two individuals - have undergone an increasing historical evolution. Indeed, the relationship between patient and doctor has evolved from a paternalistic model, in which the doctor held exclusive decision-making authority without consulting the patient, to a model of patient-centred care. This paradigm shift has led to the recognition of patients' rights as an essential element of medical ethics. The patient is no longer perceived as a passive subject receiving care, but as an autonomous individual with the right to make informed decisions about his or her health.

By protecting patients' autonomy, preserving their dignity and fostering trust between patients and healthcare professionals, these developments have helped to improve the quality of care.

Recognition of patients' rights aims to guarantee respect for human dignity and individual autonomy in the healthcare field. It is based on fundamental principles such as the right to information, informed consent and confidentiality. These rights, reinforced and institutionalized by the ethical principles of medical deontology and by their legal consecration, enable patients to make informed decisions about their care and to participate actively in their management. This approach makes a significant contribution to promoting quality care and strengthening the relationship of trust between healthcare professionals.

Knowledge of patients' rights is essential to quality medicine. This in-depth understanding can have a significant impact on the quality of patient care and, by extension, on the relationship between patient and caregiver. Indeed, it acts as a necessary counterbalance to the duties of the nursing staff, fostering a fair and respectful balance in the care relationship. What's more, mastering these standards helps prevent disputes and complaints against healthcare professionals.

Despite the importance of patients' rights, studies have revealed gaps in healthcare professionals' knowledge of medical law and ethics. Indeed, a study conducted in Nepal revealed that a significant proportion of doctors were unaware of key health ethics documents, such as the Hippocratic Oath (33% of doctors were unaware of it), the Nuremberg Code (90% of doctors were unaware of it) and the Declaration of Helsinki (85% of doctors were unaware of it)(3). These shortcomings can have a negative impact on the quality of care and the patient-caregiver relationship. It is therefore crucial to implement effective strategies to strengthen the knowledge and skills of healthcare professionals in this field.

In this work, we set ourselves the following objectives:

- Assessing healthcare professionals' knowledge of patients' rights;
- Propose a strategy to improve healthcare professionals' knowledge of patients' rights.

II. CHAPTER 2: Patients' rights

The right to health cannot be reduced to mere access to care, but encompasses the right to quality care, involving services that are efficient, safe, respectful of human dignity and adapted to the specific needs of each patient. This broader conception of the right to health underlines the importance of guaranteeing not only the availability of health services, but also their adequacy to patients' legitimate expectations and rights.

A. Right to life:

The right to life is a fundamental right that justifies the right to care. It is the primary motivation for medical conduct, obliging healthcare professionals to provide immediate assistance to sick or injured people in danger, or to ensure that they receive the necessary care. This obligation to help a person in danger, enshrined in the Hippocratic Oath and medical codes of ethics, underlines the primordial importance of human life and health.

Healthcare professionals are thus obliged to intervene quickly and effectively in emergency situations, in order to preserve the life and health of the patient. This ethical commitment to protecting and supporting individuals in the most critical moments underlines the inseparable link between the right to life and the duty to provide care.

This fundamental right to life also includes the right of every individual to have access to quality health care, without discrimination and in an equitable manner. It guarantees health protection, notably through disease prevention, health promotion and access to appropriate medical services. Thus, the right to life and the right to health are closely linked, forming a set of inalienable rights aimed at preserving the dignity and well-being of the human person.

The right to life is enshrined in several legislative texts and international legal instruments ratified by Tunisia. Article 43 of the Tunisian Constitution stipulates that: "*Every human being has the right to health. The State guarantees prevention and health care to all citizens, and provides the necessary resources to ensure the safety and quality of health services. The State guarantees free health care for people without support or with insufficient resources.*"(4)

This right is also reaffirmed in Law no. 91-63 of July 29, 1991 on health organization. Article 1 of this law states that "*Everyone has the right to protection of their health in the best possible conditions*", while article 3 affirms that "*Everyone has the right of access to preventive, curative, palliative, diagnostic and functional rehabilitation services, with or without hospitalization, in return for payment or free of charge*".(5).

The right to life raises complex ethical issues when confronted with the notion of the "right to die". Two fundamental questions emerge from this reflection: does the patient have the right to decide to end his or her own life and control his or her own death? Do they have the right to violate their physical integrity?

Although suicide is not generally criminalized, aiding suicide is often considered a reprehensible act. In Tunisia, article 206 of the Penal Code provides for penalties for those who knowingly participate in a suicide(6). This legislation aims to protect vulnerable individuals and prevent possible abuse.

However, the question of individual autonomy and respect for freedom of choice remains at the heart of the debate. Should patients in extreme suffering be granted the right to end their lives, even with the help of others? This delicate issue raises profound moral, religious and legal considerations.

In our socio-cultural and religious context, euthanasia is still considered an act of voluntary homicide punishable by death. Indeed, article 201 of the Tunisian Penal Code (CPT) stipulates that "*Anyone who, by any means whatsoever, wilfully and premeditatedly commits homicide shall be punished by death.*" (6).

Under no circumstances is a doctor authorized to perform an act aimed at helping a patient to die. When faced with a request for euthanasia, the doctor is obliged to inform the patient of his refusal. However, it is imperative for the physician to refrain from any form of therapeutic overkill, while respecting the principle of beneficence and guaranteeing the comfort and dignity of the patient at the end of life.

B. The right to healthcare :

The Tunisian Code of Medical Ethics (CDMT) explicitly emphasizes the fundamental right to quality care. This regulatory text guarantees the quality of care and medical acts through various essential provisions.

Article 32 of the Tunisian Code of Medical Ethics (CDMT) underlines the crucial commitment of the physician to elaborate his or her diagnosis with the utmost rigor, calling, if necessary, on enlightened advice and appropriate scientific methods (7). This requirement for diagnostic accuracy is crucial to the doctor's commitment to the patient, obliging him or her to provide conscientious, dedicated care based on acquired scientific data. This notion of a "contract of care" establishes an implicit agreement between patient and physician, demanding attentive care that conforms to established medical standards.

Similarly, Article 13 of the CDMT specifies that "..., *a physician must never, except in exceptional circumstances, undertake or continue care, nor formulate prescriptions in fields with which he is unfamiliar and which exceed his competence and recognized qualification.*"(7). It is therefore essential for the physician, as stipulated in Article 4 of the CDMT, not to compromise the quality of care and medical acts, except in cases of necessity justified by the interests of the patient. (7).

In addition, the right to continuity of care, enshrined in articles 37 and 38 of the CDMT, highlights the physician's obligation to ensure continuous and harmonious care for his patients. (7). The aim of this principle is to guarantee optimum quality of care, as well as sustained attention to the well-being of those being cared for, by avoiding breaks in the care trajectory. Physicians must therefore ensure the coherence and coordination of medical interventions, by monitoring patients and encouraging the transmission of relevant information between healthcare professionals.

These deontological and constitutional principles highlight the medical profession's commitment to protecting health and respecting patients' rights, while emphasizing the importance of competence, quality of care and continuity in medical practice.

C. The right to personal dignity and integrity:

The right to personal dignity and integrity, a fundamental principle of human rights, is an essential pillar of modern healthcare systems, guaranteeing quality care that respects patients' rights and freedoms.

This right implies respect for the whole person, taking into account his or her beliefs and values, alleviating suffering and protecting against unjustified harm to body and mind.

According to Article 3 of the Charter of Fundamental Rights of the European Union, everyone has the right to physical and mental integrity, and this right must be respected, protected and guaranteed. (8).

Respect for the dignity and integrity of the individual includes the fundamental right to be treated with respect, to enjoy a dignified end of life, to maintain one's dignity until death, to receive benevolent care, and to have one's integrity preserved during care. This principle also implies the patient's informed consent, respect for autonomy, confidentiality of medical data, protection of privacy and equitable access to care.

Any violation of these principles, such as lack of information, coercion into treatment, unauthorized disclosure of information, lack of respect or privacy, or discrimination, constitutes a serious attack on the patient's dignity and integrity.

These ethical and legal principles underline the importance of preserving the dignity and integrity of each individual, guaranteeing respectful care and a dignified end of life, and preventing any form of abuse or physical or moral harm.

D. Right to inviolability of the body :

The right to inviolability of the human body, enshrined in international human rights law, is a fundamental principle in Tunisia, anchored in the Constitution and national laws. Although not explicitly mentioned, article 25 of the Tunisian Constitution states that "*The State protects the dignity of the human being and his physical integrity, and prohibits moral and physical torture*".(4)thus providing a constitutional basis for the protection of physical integrity.

From a deontological point of view, article 2 of the CDMT stipulates: "*Respect for life and for the human person constitutes in all circumstances the paramount duty of the physician*".(7). Respect for this right implies the obligation to obtain the patient's consent to the act of care, except in emergencies.

Patients have the right to refuse treatment, and no action can be taken on their body without their consent. The difficulty arises when vital care is required but the patient refuses. The doctor is faced with a dilemma: between the duty to respect the patient's wishes and the obligation to respect life, and therefore the duty to help a person in danger. In this context, the doctor must provide the patient with information about the risks involved in refusing treatment.

Article 18 of Decree no. 81-1634 of 30/11/1981, setting out the general internal regulations for hospitals: "*Any patient of full age and in full possession of his or her mental faculties who wishes to leave the establishment before recovery and despite the advice of the Head of Department to the contrary, must submit a written and signed request to release the establishment from its responsibility. In the case of minors or incapacitated adults, the request in question must be made by the parents or legal guardian.*(9).

Thus, respect for the inviolability of the body is essential, except in the case of legitimate exceptions provided for by law. Indeed, patients suffering from certain transmissible diseases (HIV infection, cholera, etc.) may be obliged to undergo regular treatment, and to provide proof of this by producing medical certificates on dates set by the health authority. (10).

E. The right to non-discrimination :

Equality of rights is affirmed by the Universal Declaration of Human Rights, which prohibits all forms of discrimination.

This principle is enshrined in various international instruments, notably the International Covenant on Economic, Social and Cultural Rights (article 12), which recognizes the right of everyone to physical and mental health, as well as to preventive, curative and rehabilitative health care (11).

Article 1 of the Patient's Charter states that everyone has the right to the protection of his or her health in the best possible conditions, without any discrimination based on religion, sex, race, age or socio-economic status.(12). Article 3 of the CDMT stipulates that *"The physician must treat all his patients with the same conscience, without discrimination"*.(7).

Respect for the right to non-discrimination in healthcare is essential to ensure equitable access to care and the promotion of health for all. This is a major challenge that requires the collective mobilization of governments, healthcare system players and civil society.

F. Right to privacy :

Respect for the right to confidentiality is the cornerstone of medicine and the basis of the patient-caregiver relationship, protected by deontological and legal provisions: "*No medicine without confidence, no confidence without trust*". (13). Physicians demonstrate their respect for patients by protecting their confidentiality.

The right to confidentiality is extended by a right to intimacy and a right to privacy. Physicians must examine their patients in conditions that respect their privacy. He must also ensure that the confidentiality of his correspondence is respected.

This right applies to all aspects of patient care, as well as to all medical and non-medical information that comes to the physician's knowledge in the exercise of his or her profession. Article 8 of the CDMT stipulates that "*all doctors are bound by professional secrecy, unless otherwise provided by law*".(7). The physician must ensure that his assistants are informed of their obligations in terms of professional secrecy and comply with them, as stated in article 9 of the CDMT: "*The physician must ensure that the persons who assist him in his work are informed of their obligations in terms of professional secrecy and comply with them*".(7).

However, there are limits to the right to confidentiality. Established in the interest of the patient, the rule of medical confidentiality can be lifted when a higher interest, that of the community, justifies it. The law thus specifies the situations in which doctors are obliged or authorized to divulge information that is normally confidential (legal exceptions to medical confidentiality: notification of births, deaths, industrial accidents and occupational illnesses, reporting of child abuse, etc.).

Breach of professional secrecy is punishable under article 254 of the Tunisian Penal Code: "*Doctors, surgeons and other health workers, pharmacists, midwives and all other persons who, by virtue of their status or profession, are entrusted with secrets, will have revealed these secrets, except in cases where the law obliges or authorizes them to act as whistle-blowers*", *are liable to six months' imprisonment and a fine of one hundred and twenty dinars.*(6).

G. Right to information :

The patient's right to medical information is a fundamental pillar of the medical contract and the relationship of trust between doctor and patient. It is of the utmost importance, and has moral, ethical and legal foundations. It is justified by the patient's right to autonomy.

Before any medical intervention, it is essential to provide clear, fair information adapted to the individual's ability to understand, in order to obtain his or her free and informed consent.(12).

As a fundamental element of the healing process, this information is a prerequisite for informed consent, adherence and active participation by the patient in his or her own treatment.

A clear understanding of the various diagnoses, objectives, nature and course of the proposed care, as well as the necessary preventive procedures, facilitates an autonomous and informed decision by the patient, thus strengthening the relationship of trust between the healthcare professional and the person being cared for.(12).

The medical record must state that the patient has been informed of all the necessary data and information referred to above.

In the case of minors and incapacitated adults, the information must be communicated to their legal guardian. In the event of a serious or fatal prognosis, the information may be withheld from the patient. It may, however, be disclosed to the immediate family, unless the patient has expressly forbidden such disclosure or designated the third parties to whom it is to be communicated (article 36 of the CDMT).(7).

H. Consent to care :

By virtue of the fundamental principle of the inviolability of the human body, any medical procedure or treatment requires the prior consent of the person concerned. Freedom of consent is a fundamental human right. Ethical and professional standards in the healthcare field emphasize the importance of respecting patients' autonomy in decisions concerning their health, and of obtaining their informed consent in the doctor-patient relationship.

Except in cases where the patient suffers from an illness that alters his or her capacity for discernment, all patients should always be able to give the doctor their informed consent before any medical examination.

In most cases, consent is given verbally. However, in specific situations, written consent is required by Tunisian law. This is particularly the case for procedures such as organ removal from the living, drug experimentation or medically assisted procreation.

Although consent is generally required, there are exceptions in specific situations. In medical emergencies, where the patient is in critical condition and unable to give consent, healthcare professionals are empowered to take measures necessary to save the patient's life or prevent serious damage to health. Similarly, in the case of transmissible diseases or serious mental disorders, doctors may act without the patient's explicit consent in order to protect public health or prevent harm to the patient him/herself. For example, an individual suffering from a communicable disease who is aware of his or her condition, refuses treatment and knowingly continues to contaminate those around him or her, may be subject to coercive measures to preserve public health.

I. Right to free choice of caregiver and access to medical records :

The right to free choice of healthcare provider is guaranteed in the private sector. In the public sector, this right is not absolute, as the patient is referred to a whole health care team. However, depending on the organization of the service, patients may be granted the right to be treated by the doctor or nurse of their choice.

The right of access to medical records is an essential right for patients, guaranteeing transparency and protection of their medical information, as well as continuity of care.

In the public sector, the medical file remains the property of the establishment, in accordance with article 72 of Decree 81-1634 of 30/11/1981 on the general internal regulations of hospitals, which stipulates that " *staff must supervise the keeping of departmental documents and draw up patients' medical files in particular. These records are and remain the property of the establishment*".(9).

According to the Ministry of Health decree of May 28, 2001, approving the specifications for private health establishments, medical records must be kept in the establishment's archives. A copy must be issued at the request of the patient, his legal guardian, his attending physician or his beneficiaries. (14).

In addition, medical imaging and biological analysis documents must be provided on request. This provision ensures that patients have access to their medical records, enabling them to consult information concerning their health and share it with the healthcare professionals involved in their care.

This right strengthens the relationship of trust between the patient and the medical profession, and promotes better understanding and informed decision-making about their health.

J. Right to compensation :

The patient has the right to civil compensation for any damage suffered as a result of medical care, whether or not there has been medical negligence. This principle implies that any person who suffers damage caused by medical malpractice or by a malfunction in the healthcare system can obtain compensation for the harm suffered.

For medical liability to be incurred, three cumulative conditions must be met:

- A fault: A fault may be committed by a doctor, a healthcare professional, a healthcare facility or a healthcare service. This fault may consist of a diagnostic error, a treatment error, a lack of information, an absence of informed consent...
- Damage: Damage can be physical, psychological or material. It may involve bodily injury, disability, cosmetic damage, mental suffering, health expenses, loss of earnings, etc.

- A causal link between the fault and the damage: It must be shown that the damage was directly caused by the fault committed.

This is a legal and ethical obligation for healthcare professionals, who must compensate for damage caused by medical errors or breaches of duty of care. This right guarantees the protection of patients' rights and the responsibility of healthcare professionals in dealing with personal injury.

III. CHAPTER 3: Assessing the knowledge of medical staff

A. Materials and methods:

1. Type of study :

This is a descriptive and analytical cross-sectional study, including healthcare professionals working in the public sector (university hospitals (CHU), regional hospitals (HR)).

2. Study population :

Our survey was carried out among healthcare professionals working in public establishments.

a) Inclusion criteria:

Healthcare professionals include pharmacists, dentists, physicians and medical residents of all specialties working in public hospitals, whether university centers or regional hospitals.

b) 2.2 Non-inclusion criteria :

- Doctors specializing in forensic medicine.
- Doctors working in the private sector.

3. Data collection :

Data were collected via a pre-established French-language questionnaire with two themes: the first included questions relating to the domain of patients' rights and health ethics , and the second dealt with a more specific theme relating to the health rights of people deprived of their liberty .

Persons deprived of their liberty" means persons under the control of the law, deprived of their right to liberty for a specified period because of acts for which they have been convicted. (15). Different terms are used to designate different groups of people deprived of their liberty: "prévenus", "en cours de jugement", "incarcérés" or "détenus".(15).

The questionnaire consists of three parts. The first part includes questions designed to specify the participants' profile without revealing their identity (age, gender, grade, specialty, place of practice and whether they have attended a conference on the subject). The second part consists of single- or multiple-choice, closed-response questions designed to assess participants' level of knowledge of patients' rights and medical ethics in general. The third part includes questions on the health rights of people deprived of their liberty.

The choice of questions was based on practical clinical situations faced by practitioners in their day-to-day practice, to highlight the seriousness of the ethical issues at stake and the medico-legal consequences that flow from them.

The clinical cases dealt with the following themes: information and consent, medical confidentiality, non-assistance to a person in danger, choice of doctor and access to medical records, medical research, end of life (Appendices).

4. Data analysis :

Data analysis was performed using Statistical Package for Social Sciences (SPSS) for Windows, version 21.0.

5. Descriptive section

For a descriptive study, two new variables were created: "Score 1" and "score2", containing the score awarded for the second and third parts of the questionnaire for each participant (1 point for each correct answer to each question).

Thus, to increase the power of our analysis, we identified three groups of participants:

→ For the second part of the questionnaire :

- Those with "Low knowledge" < or equal to 10

- Those with "Average knowledge" 11-20

- Those with "Good Knowledge" > 20

→ For the third part of the questionnaire :

- Those with "Low knowledge" < or equal to 5.

- Those with "Average knowledge" 6-11.

- Those with "Good Knowledge" > 12.

Qualitative variables were expressed as frequencies, quantitative variables as averages.

6. **Analytical part**

For the purposes of univariate analysis, participants with "Average Knowledge" and those with "Low Knowledge" were grouped together into a single "Poor Knowledge" group.

We then performed a univariate analysis to identify the factors associated with poor knowledge.

Percentage comparisons were made by Pearson's Chi 2 test if all theoretical numbers were greater than or equal to 5, and by Fisher's test otherwise.

The statistical significance level was set at 0.05.

7. Ethical considerations :

This work presents no conflict of interest. The questionnaire was filled in voluntarily and anonymously by the participants after clear information on the purpose of the work.

B. Results of medical staff knowledge assessment

1. Part 1: assessment of medical staff's knowledge of health law and ethics

Out of 384 questionnaires distributed, 243 were fully completed, giving a response rate of 63.28%. The age of questionnaire participants ranged from 26 to 54 years, with an average of 32.73 ± 5.61 years. In this study, women predominated, with a sex ratio of 0.64.

In addition, almost all participating physicians (96.3%) stated that they had not attended a conference on medical law and health ethics. According to the score used, the majority of participants had an average level of knowledge

(Table I). Participants with "Poor Knowledge" accounted for 60.9% (this is obtained by summing the percentages of "Average Knowledge" and "Poor Knowledge" participants).

Table I: Participants' knowledge levels

Knowledge	**Workforce**	**Percentage (%)**
Good	95	39,1
Average	167	60,5
Low	01	0,4

a) Consent, information :

The first question concerned consent to care. Almost all participants (99.6%) felt that clear and fair information was necessary to obtain consent to care before any action was taken.

Eighty-two percent ticked the box "Consent must be given in writing", and 68.7% said that in most cases it is given orally.

Four percent of respondents considered that the husband's consent is obligatory in the case of a voluntary interruption of pregnancy.

With regard to information, 22.6% of participants felt that it was compulsory, even in emergencies. Two point five percent of participants replied that they could withhold information about a transmissible disease such as AIDS from the patient because of the psychological repercussions. Almost half (55.6%) of the respondents included in this study said that a serious prognosis could be withheld from the patient.

b) The right to choose a doctor and access medical records :

For this question, the correct answer is "You inform her that she will be operated on by the surgeon according to the organization of the service and the availability of surgeons".

Whereas 26.3% of doctors surveyed stated that patients do not have the right to choose their surgeon, regardless of whether they are hospitalized in a private or public hospital.

Under what circumstances can a person be denied access to his or her medical file? Does he or she have the right to receive a copy of the discharge summary to ensure optimal continuity of care?

For continuity of care in a polyclinic, 41.2% of participants believe that patients have the right to have their entire medical file.

c) *Medical confidentiality :*

➢ Medical confidentiality / minors

For the question relating to medical confidentiality concerning a minor, if a minor objects to the transmission of information concerning him or her to his or her parents, 37.9% (n=92) of participants expressed their agreement not to communicate this information to the minor's parents (for his or her physical welfare).

- Reporting to the authorities by nursing staff :

Regarding the question on reporting by medical staff to the authorities, 97.9% of participating doctors ticked "report violence against women", 98.4% ticked "report child abuse " and 93.4% ticked "report a crime in the making". Twenty point six percent ticked "report a crime already committed". Also 8.6% of respondents said they would report a criminal offence confessed to by a patient consulting them.

For the question on child abuse, the situation of an indication for urgent hospitalization of an abused child was posed, but the father refused and just asked for a medical prescription. Only 12.8% of the doctors questioned ticked the wrong box "Respect the wishes of the legal guardian".

- Medical confidentiality and communicable diseases

Only 2.5% of healthcare professionals surveyed agreed to inform the spouse of an HIV patient about his or her condition, and 5.5% did not know the appropriate attitude in this case.

d) Drug research

Seven percent of the doctors who took part in the present study believe that pregnant women could be candidates for drug research.

Concerning consent for all stages of research and adverse effects, 36.2% of doctors surveyed believe that consent is given orally.

e) Non-assistance to a person in danger:

In the distributed questionnaire, we proposed the following situation: a patient with multiple pathologies and terminal cancer is brought to the emergency department in a coma requiring intubation, but the doctor refuses to intervene, believing it to be a hopeless case. The question asked whether participants agreed with the doctor (yes or no), and 33.3% of them ticked "Yes". Next, we asked if the doctor's responsibility was engaged, and 11.9% of participants ticked "No".

f) End of life

Concerning the question posed by a patient suffering from a terminal neoplastic disease who, while hospitalized, asks his doctor to put an end to his suffering by helping him to die with dignity, 2.5% of doctors questioned expressed their approval.

2. Part 2: Assessment of medical staff's knowledge of the health rights of persons deprived of their liberty

a) Characteristics of the study population :

The majority of participants (97.2%) in the present study had not attended a conference concerning the rights of people deprived of their liberty.

Only one participant managed to answer all the questions correctly. All participants answered only two questions correctly. Table II shows the distribution of medical staff according to their level of knowledge in the field of the right to health of individuals deprived of liberty.

Table II: Distribution according to participants' level of knowledge

Knowledge	*Workforce*	*Percentage*
Good	41	16,9%
Average	189	77,7%
Low	13	5,4%

b) Consent to care :

Almost two-thirds of participants (69.4%) felt that it is necessary to obtain the consent of a patient deprived of liberty before carrying out a physical examination or any act of care. Whereas thirty point six percent thought that permission must be obtained from security officers to examine and treat a patient in police custody .

c) Medical confidentiality :

Only almost half the participants (58.3%) believe that doctors should not pass on information about the state of health of a patient deprived of liberty to police officers.

A quarter of the participants felt that a past offence committed by the patient should be reported to the authorities, while 41.7% felt that a "crime already committed" admitted by the patient during the interview should not be reported.

d) Non-assistance to a person in peril :

In this context, we proposed the situation of a capital prisoner, diagnosed as positive for SARS-Covid-19, presenting with an altered general condition and signs of respiratory distress. The prison doctor refused to intervene for fear of running the risk of contamination by a murderer. The question asked was whether the participants agreed with the doctor's attitude ("yes" or "no") and whether the doctor could be held criminally liable in this case.

All participants disapproved of the doctor's attitude. Eighty-three of those questioned assumed that the doctor would be held criminally liable.

e) Drug research in persons deprived of liberty :

Half the participants thought that people deprived of their liberty could not be candidates for clinical trials in medical research, while 22.2% said they could take part.

C. Discussion of results:

1. Factors influencing the level of knowledge:

The inadequacy of participants' knowledge, whether declarative, procedural or conditional, in the field of health ethics and patients' rights, is confirmed both by our study and by data in the literature (3,16,17).

Of the healthcare professionals included in our study, only 3.7% had attended conferences on medical law and health ethics. This figure is in line with findings in the literature: a study conducted in Nigeria in 2012 found that 24.7% of doctors surveyed said they had attended conferences on these topics (18).

In our study, 60.9% of participants had an insufficient level of knowledge. A 2016 study of 200 doctors in India by G. Venkat Rao et al. found that 84 interns (70%) and 32 post-graduate doctors (40%) had no adequate knowledge to handle medico-legal cases independently(19).

This lack of awareness is due to a lack of training among healthcare professionals, but also to initial university training that focuses too much on theoretical instruction. For example, in a study carried out in the USA in 2020, 46% of gynecology-obstetrics residents who responded to the questionnaire stated that forensic training was provided informally or by observing colleagues, and 15% said they had received no education in this area at all (20).

It is fundamental and essential that doctors are aware of these decision-making tools in order to protect the trust they have with their patients as part of the care pact. A study carried out in Nepal on the importance of ethics in the medical field showed that a large majority (91.3%) of participants considered it to be very important(21).

2. Right to information :

Doctors have a legal and ethical obligation to inform their patients in a fair, clear and appropriate manner about their state of health and the investigations and care they are proposing, whatever the medical procedure envisaged, whether therapeutic (preventive or curative) or not.

In accordance with the patient charter, doctors are exempt from their obligation to inform patients only in very specific cases:

- In proven emergency situations, when any delay in treatment could seriously compromise the patient's health.
- When the patient explicitly refuses to be informed, except in the case of a transmissible disease
- When the patient's state of health makes it impossible to provide clear and appropriate information.(12)

Our study revealed that 2.5% of participating doctors were willing to withhold information from a patient suffering from a transmissible disease. This result is similar to that of the study carried out by Aissaoui.A et al. which revealed that 18% of doctors surveyed were prepared to withhold this type of information from their patients (23).

Under article 6 of Law 92-71 of July 27, 1992, amended in 2007, on transmissible diseases (10), patients suffering from such diseases must be informed of their diagnosis. This obligation is designed to prevent the transmission of the disease to the patient's family and friends. The doctor must inform the patient of the nature of the disease, its possible consequences and the risks of contamination if preventive measures are not taken. Failure to comply with these provisions may result in penal sanctions. (10).

On the other hand, 44.4% of participants stressed that a serious prognosis should not be withheld from the patient, while 8.6% indicated that they would not disclose this information to a close family member. Research by Yuxiu Liu et al. in 2018 highlighted that many patients expressed a wish to be informed of a terminal illness diagnosis (91.9% vs. 53.2%, P <0.01)(25).

In accordance with article 36 of the Code of Medical Ethics (CDM), in certain exceptional situations where the prognosis is bleak or fatal, the doctor may exceptionally withhold this information from the patient. However, he or she must then inform the immediate family, unless the patient has previously prohibited such disclosure or designated the third parties to whom it is to be communicated.(7).

The aim of this provision is to protect the patient from being told too abruptly of a fatal prognosis, while respecting his or her right to information and enabling his or her family to be informed in order to provide the best possible support. But it remains a limited exception, the principle being that the doctor must inform the patient in good faith of his or her state of health.

3. Right to consent :

In accordance with the principle of inviolability of the human body, all medical procedures require the prior consent of the patient. Freedom of consent is a fundamental right that ethical and professional standards in the healthcare sector emphasize as essential to respecting patients' autonomy in decisions concerning their health.

To this end, doctors have a duty to clearly inform patients of their state of health, the procedures envisaged and their consequences, so that they can give informed consent. This right to information is essential to enable patients to exercise autonomy in decisions concerning their health.

In the present study, 80.2% of the doctors who completed the questionnaire thought that consent to care should be in writing. This result is similar to that of a study carried out in India in 2017 by Mahesh Jambure et al. (22)which showed that 62 (62.0%) of interns and 75 (93.75%) post-graduate doctors responded that the best type of medical consent is written and informed consent (22).

These attitudes do not comply with the Tunisian legal framework. In fact, consent to care is traditionally given orally, except for certain procedures such as organ removal from a living person, biomedical experimentation and reproductive medicine procedures (12,23).

In the case of a minor patient, the care contract is drawn up with his or her legal guardian. The guardian must be present when the minor is examined, and must give his or her consent for any diagnostic or therapeutic procedure.

Nevertheless, 4.9% of participants admitted to treating a minor without obtaining parental consent. A study conducted by Aissaoui.A et al in 2018 revealed that 18% of participants also agreed to provide care to a minor without obtaining parental consent (24). A study by Gupta G et al. found that 59.1% of doctors surveyed said they would obtain consent from the legal guardian before performing a tooth extraction on a 17-year-old patient (25).

For detainees and prisoners, although they are deprived of their liberty, they retain all their rights as human beings, with the exception of those they have lost as a result of their deprivation of liberty. These rights are protected by the provisions of the Constitution, which stipulates that "*Every prisoner has the right to humane treatment that preserves his or her dignity*" (article 36)(4).

In our survey, 69.4% of participants felt that the detainee's consent should be obtained for the physical examination and before any act of care.

Except in cases where the subject suffers from an illness impairing his or her capacity for discernment, the person deprived of liberty should always be able to give the doctor informed consent prior to any medical examination. Furthermore, any derogation from the principle of freedom of consent should be established by law and follow the same principles that apply to the general population.

Thirty point six percent of the participants in our study believe that permission must be obtained from security officers to examine and treat a patient in police custody. This attitude is at odds with Nelson Mandela's rules, which state that "*clinical decisions can only be made by responsible health professionals*" and "*cannot be rejected or ignored by non-medical prison staff*" (26). It is important to note that the health care of the person deprived of liberty is based solely on medical criteria established by the health professional, remembering that according to article 11 of the code of medical ethics "*The doctor may not alienate his professional independence in any form whatsoever.*"(7).

4. Right to choose a doctor and to access medical records :

In this study, 26.3% of doctors surveyed indicated that patients cannot choose their surgeon, regardless of whether they are hospitalized in a private or public hospital.

In accordance with the European Patient's Charter, every individual has the right to select his or her healthcare team and to choose freely among various treatment procedures, based on adequate information. (8).

Free choice of healthcare provider is a right that is fully guaranteed to patients in the private healthcare sector. In the public sector, however, there are limits to this principle. Patients generally turn to a healthcare team as a whole, rather than to an individual professional.

Nevertheless, depending on the internal organization of each public health establishment, it is sometimes possible for patients to obtain the favor of being treated by the doctor or nurse of their choice. This right remains less absolute than in the private sector, where patients are free to consult the healthcare professional of their choice without restriction.

As far as hospital medical records are concerned, the record (container) is the property of the hospital, while its contents belong to the patient, who may dispose of them. On discharge, a copy of the hospitalization summary is given to the patient (patient's right) to ensure continuity of care.

5. Medical confidentiality :

Medical secrecy (SM) covers all information entrusted to us, as well as anything seen, heard, understood or even interpreted by the doctor.

➤ Medical confidentiality / minors :

In the case of a minor patient, the physician has a legal and ethical obligation to inform the parents or legal guardians and obtain their consent before any medical intervention. However, in certain special cases, such as that of a pregnant 17-year-old minor, the doctor may be faced with an ethical dilemma. On the one hand, he must, in principle, inform the parents and obtain their consent. On the other hand, he must also protect the minor from potential violence from those around him, and act in his best interests. In this situation, the doctor must discerningly assess the risks and benefits for the minor patient, giving priority to his or her protection and well-being. He may consider obtaining the minor's consent alone, if the latter is capable of giving consent and if informing the parents could seriously harm him. In this case, however, the physician must carefully record his or her reasoning in the medical file.

A study carried out in 2020 in Belgrade, Serbia, by Vida Jeremic Stojkovic et al. (27) studying medical confidentiality in the face of adolescents using several scales, showed that out of a total of 20 items, one did not show significant factorial saturation and was excluded from the scale. This item was "The family should be involved in making important decisions about the health of all its members." (27)

- <u>Medical confidentiality (SM)/Reporting to the authorities</u>

According to article 8 of the CDMT, "*all doctors are bound by professional secrecy, unless otherwise stipulated by law*". (7).

The purpose of SM is to protect a private interest, that of the patient. The private interest becomes blurred when the public interest is at stake, hence the legal derogations to SM. These derogations are dictated by law. It should be remembered that these exceptions are provided for in Art 254 CPT, which ends with: "*... except where the law obliges or authorizes them to act as whistleblowers*". (6) and Art 8 of the CDMT: "*... unless otherwise provided by law*".(7).

All doctors are therefore obliged to declare the fact discovered by the SM to the authority provided for in this derogation. Failure to report is punishable by law.

In our survey, 20.6% answered that they would report a crime that had already been committed, which is wrong because a crime that has already been committed, such as an act of terrorism, is covered by medical confidentiality. Unlike a crime in the making, in this case the doctor is obliged to report it.

Indeed, according to Art 37 of Law 2015-26 of August 07 relating to the fight against terrorism and the repression of money laundering: "*is guilty of a terrorist offence and punishable by one to five years' imprisonment and a fine of five thousand dinars whoever, even if bound by professional secrecy, fails to report to the competent authorities, without delay and within the limits of the acts of which he has become aware, facts, information or intelligence concerning the commission of terrorist offences provided for by this law or their possible commission."* (28)

"The provisions of the preceding paragraph do not apply to ascendants, descendants or spouses.

Lawyers and doctors *are also excepted with regard to secrets of which they have become aware during or on the occasion of the exercise of their mission. Also excluded are journalists, in accordance with the provisions of Decree-Law no. 2011-115 of November 2, 2011, on freedom of the press, printing and publishing.* (29) ".

These exceptions do not extend to information of which they have become aware, and the reporting of which to the authorities would have made it possible to prevent the commission of terrorist offences in the future.

Child abuse also constitutes a legal exception to medical confidentiality. Article 31 of the child protection code (law 95-92) establishes an obligation to report any physical or moral abuse of a child by a doctor*: "Any person, including those bound by professional secrecy, is duty-bound to report to the child protection officer anything likely* *to constitute a threat to the child's health, or to his or her physical or moral integrity (child abuse, sexual exploitation of children, whether boys or girls)*".(30).

- <u>Medical confidentiality and communicable diseases :</u>

With regard to transmissible diseases, all doctors must declare the confirmed diagnosis of a transmissible disease to the patient and to the health authorities.

Article 7 of Law 92-71 of July 27, 1992, as supplemented and amended by Law 2007-12 of February 12, 2007 on transmissible diseases, requires any doctor or biologist who has diagnosed or become aware of the transmissible diseases listed in article 3 of the law and set by order of the Ministry of Public Health (MSP), to declare them to the health authorities, regardless of his or her status or mode of practice.(10).

A study carried out in Brazil in 2021 by Gabriela Kato Lettieri et al. (31) showed that according to the CRM-PR (the Regional Council of Medicine of the State of Paraná), doctors may not respect medical secrecy for the collective well-being. Such notification is a legal obligation that justifies the derogation of medical confidentiality (31).

A 2012 study in Belgium by Bjorn Ketels et al. (32) showed that the doctor must inform the partner of a person with a sexually transmitted disease about his or her illness, so as not to commit the offence under Article 422bis of the Belgian Penal Code relating to culpable abstention. This seems to apply to both HIV and other STIs. This position has been partially accepted by the ethics authorities, at least as far as HIV is concerned, since they have provided "permission" to inform the partner if necessary. (32).

The question of a wife requesting information about her husband's state of health while in hospital for treatment of HIV infection raises a complex ethical dilemma. On the one hand, the patient has a fundamental right to the confidentiality of his medical information. On the other, the doctor has a duty of non-maleficence that could oblige him or her to inform the partner exposed to the risk of contamination.

There is no simple solution to this conflict between respecting patient privacy and protecting the spouse's health. It requires careful consideration of the ethical principles involved and the potential consequences of each decision. The doctor must carefully weigh up the various interests involved before making a decision.

- Medical confidentiality and persons deprived of their liberty :

Medical confidentiality must be respected for detainees in accordance with the same legal provisions as for free persons. All medical procedures are carried out in the absence of any prison or judicial personnel.

However, in certain situations where security concerns need to be taken into account, it may be necessary to allow consultations to take place under the visual supervision of prison staff, while preserving auditory confidentiality.(15). According to the United Nations Bangkok Rules, medical staff should be the only ones present during medical examinations, unless the doctor deems the circumstances to be exceptional, or requests the presence of a member of prison staff for security reasons, or if the prisoner expressly so requests(33).

In our study, more than half the participants (58.3%) felt that the doctor should not divulge information about the state of health of a patient deprived of liberty to police officers.

Medical confidentiality is enforceable against any third party, including the authorities, even if that authority is itself bound by professional secrecy. It covers all aspects of health care for persons deprived of their liberty, as well as all information, whether medical or not, which comes to the knowledge of the doctor in the exercise of his profession. This is why the Nelson Mandela Rules (RNM) insist that "all medical examinations must be carried out in complete confidentiality", and more generally establish "the confidentiality of medical information, except in the event of a real and imminent threat to the patient or others". (26).

6. Drug research :

For many years now, scientific experimentation on human beings has been the subject of constant interest from legislators and regulators, with the aim of preventing abuses and guaranteeing respect for the fundamental rights and well-being of individuals.

Tunisia has seen a legal evolution in the regulation of clinical trials. The modalities for medical or scientific experimentation of medicines intended for human medicine are defined in accordance with Decree no. 2014-3657 of October 3, 2014(34)amending and supplementing decree no. 90-1401 of September 3, 1990, which specifies that only adults (aged 18 and over) who possess full mental and legal capacity, and who give their written consent, may be subject to experimentation. Consent must be free, informed, revocable and continuous.

For illiterate volunteers, consent is given in the presence of a support person of their choice, who has no interest in the experiment.

Healthy volunteers may not take part in more than two experiments per year, separated by a minimum period of four months from the date of completion of the previous experiment.

Respect for individuals in biomedical research is based on a dual moral duty: on the one hand, to respect the autonomy of participants, and on the other, to protect those whose autonomy is developing, hindered or diminished.

Participants must be given full, comprehensible and appropriate information on the objectives, procedures and risks of the research, so that they can make an informed decision. Their consent must be given voluntarily, without any form of coercion or pressure.

What's more, consent must be a dynamic process, with participants able to withdraw it at any time if they wish, without having to justify themselves.

In our study, we found that 36.2% of the doctors surveyed believed that the participant's consent to the various stages of the research and to potential adverse effects could be given verbally. However, it is important to stress that Tunisian regulations require that consent be obtained in writing for any medical or scientific experiment involving drugs intended for human medicine. Indeed, the Ministry of Public Health established a model informed consent form by decree in 2015 to provide a framework for this practice.

A study conducted in Nepal in 2015 (21) highlighted that the vast majority of participating physicians (87.0%) were involved in research involving human subjects. In this context, 82.6% of them obtained written informed consent in the research process. These results underline the importance of respecting ethical and legal standards for informed consent in medical research.

In Tunisia, regulations prohibit drug research on pregnant and breast-feeding women, without distinction. In Mexico, however, a more nuanced approach is adopted. Before conducting research involving pregnant women, it is essential to clearly define whether the main object of the study is the woman herself or the developing foetus. In addition, a distinction is made between therapeutic research, aimed at improving maternal and/or fetal health, and non-therapeutic research, whose aim is to contribute to the advancement of scientific knowledge. This differentiation makes it possible to more accurately assess the potential risks and benefits for pregnant women and the fetus, and to adapt protocols accordingly. (35).

The Colorado Multiple Institutional Review Board (COMIRB) declared in March 2022 that according to the U.S. Food and Drug

Administration, pregnant women are excluded from drug research (36,37).

Minors and people with mental disabilities may be included in clinical trials for therapeutic purposes specific to their medical conditions or disabilities. In such cases, the informed, free and written consent of the legal guardian is mandatory.

People deprived of their liberty are at the heart of the ethical debate surrounding their involvement in medical research. The main question concerns their ability to give genuinely free consent, without being subjected to any pressure linked to their situation of detention.

In the present study, 52.8% of participants thought that people deprived of their liberty should not be candidates for clinical trials in the context of medical research.

The Nelson Mandela Rules state that "*prisoners may be permitted, if they give their free and informed consent, in accordance with applicable law, to participate in clinical trials and other medical research organized in society if there is expected to be a significant direct benefit to their health...*"(26).

As a result, an extremely cautious approach must be adopted when it comes to medical experimentation involving persons deprived of their liberty, considered as "*vulnerable persons in need of special protection*", according to the Declarations of Helsinki repeatedly revised by the World Medical Association (38).

All international and national ethical standards applicable to experimentation on human beings stress the principle of respect for human autonomy and dignity, as well as the obligation to obtain the individual's voluntary, informed and long-term consent. According to article 7 of the International Covenant on Economic, Social and Cultural Rights: "... *it is forbidden to subject a person without his free consent to medical or scientific experimentation*"(11).

Consequently, great care must be taken when involving an individual deprived of his or her liberty in a medical research protocol, ensuring that all legal and ethical obligations are respected, in particular respect for their autonomy. Under no circumstances should participation in a medical research protocol result in physical injury, mental suffering or other damage to the participant's health. Any violation of ethical standards is considered an attack on human integrity and falls within the scope of torture and ill-treatment.

7. Non-assistance to a person in danger :

Failure to render assistance is culpable when it is committed voluntarily, even if there is no intention to cause harm. The doctor's intervention is not conditioned by its effectiveness. It is the will to help that is more important than the result of the help itself. Doctors guilty of wrongful abstention are liable to criminal and civil prosecution, as well as disciplinary action. Penal sanctions are severe (imprisonment and fine). The provisions of art. 53 of the CPT (lowering penalties below the legal minimum) are not applicable to the offence of culpable abstention.

The doctor may also be ordered to pay compensation to the patient or his dependents. A civil judgment can only be handed down if there is proof of fault on the part of the doctor (non-assistance to a person in danger), of damage to the patient (death or bodily harm) and of a causal relationship between the two.

The guilty doctor is also liable to disciplinary action, which may be taken by the Ordre des

Médecins and by his or her employer (Ministry of Health, administration). The sanction imposed by the CNOM can range from a reprimand to dismissal.

For the vignette of a patient with terminal cancer, brought to the ER in a coma, who requires urgent care, but the doctor refuses to intervene because it's a hopeless case, 33.3% of participants adopted the same attitude. What's more, 11.9% felt that the doctor's responsibility was not engaged in this situation.

On the other hand, when caring for a patient deprived of liberty, doctors' ethical obligations are governed by the principle of equivalence of care. Article 3 of the CDMT stipulates: "*Physicians must treat all their patients with the same conscience, without discrimination of any kind*".(7). The physician is obliged to use all possible means to preserve the patient's life: "*Respect for life and the human person constitutes the physician's primary duty in all circumstances*" (article 2).(7).

Law no. 2001-52 of May 14, 2001 on the organization of prisons states in its first article that all persons deprived of their liberty "*shall benefit from medical and psychological assistance*" and that prison conditions must "*ensure the physical and moral integrity of the prisoner*". (39).

IV. CHAPTER 4: Recommendations

We propose measures to improve doctors' declarative, procedural and conditional knowledge of patients' rights and health ethics, focusing on three main areas.

The first is to strengthen doctors' declarative knowledge by harmonizing and enhancing university teaching in medical law and health ethics, and by improving their understanding of the major ethical principles underlying medical practice.

The second is to improve doctors' procedural and conditional knowledge. We recommend that students be given greater access to internships in forensic medicine departments and patients' rights units, bearing in mind the limitations of the small number of facilities compared with the large number of students to be trained, as well as the organization of student working groups, supervised by experts in medical law and medical ethics, to work on concrete clinical cases from hospital practice.

Finally, the 3rd axis will focus on the creation of a Patients' Rights Committee within the hospital. The main roles of this committee will be to

- Awareness-raising and training of healthcare staff in the area of patients' rights through the organization of practical and periodic training in this field.

- Helping doctors to make the right decisions whenever they encounter difficulties.

Conciliation between the various parties involved in the event of healthcare-related damage.

- Supporting changes in the healthcare system while respecting users' rights.

We also offer a number of internationally and nationally validated recommendations for the examination of patients deprived of their liberty, designed to ensure respect for the fundamental human rights of persons deprived of their liberty. Here are the main conditions to be respected when examining patients deprived of their liberty:

Respect for human dignity and non-discrimination: every individual, whatever their status, is entitled to respect for their dignity, and must not be discriminated against because of their situation in detention.

Independence and impartiality: doctors must enjoy complete independence from police and prison authorities. His clinical decisions and all other assessments relating to the health of detainees must be based solely on strictly medical criteria.

Medical secrecy and confidentiality: Medical examinations must take place in environments that guarantee the confidentiality of discussions and medical information. All information declared by patients must be confidential, except in cases where there is an imminent risk to the safety of the detainee or others.

Informed consent: Persons deprived of their liberty must be informed of the nature and purpose of medical examinations, and given the opportunity to give or refuse their consent, except in cases of medical emergency.

Unhindered access: Health professionals must have unhindered access to prisoners to conduct appropriate examinations.

A thorough examination: The physician must take a careful history and perform a complete examination encompassing all aspects of physical and mental health, including medical history and care needs. He must evaluate the various therapeutic options, draw up a treatment proposal, discuss it with the patient and obtain his consent. The choice of treatment is based exclusively on medical considerations, and is therefore a purely scientific decision.

Any traces of violence observed on a detainee during a medical examination must be duly recorded.

<u>Appropriate medical care</u>: Healthcare professionals must provide medical care that conforms to best practices and recognized medical standards.

<u>Proper documentation</u>: The results of medical examinations must be carefully documented, including diagnoses, recommended treatments and prescribed medications, to ensure ongoing medical follow-up.

<u>Prevention of torture and inhuman or degrading treatment</u> : Health professionals must report any cases of mistreatment, negligence or abuse observed during the examination of detainees.

V. CHAPTER 5: Conclusion s

The right to health and patients' rights are inseparable concepts, which help to promote humanized medicine that respects human dignity.

Practicing physicians' knowledge of legal and medico-legal concepts relating to patients' rights and health ethics varies, which can have an impact on the quality of care and the doctor-patient relationship.

The aim of this study was to assess doctors' practical knowledge of these essential subjects. The study revealed shortcomings in doctors' declarative, procedural and conditional knowledge of patients' rights, confirming the data in the literature. However, it seems essential that doctors should be aware of these decision-making tools, especially those who enjoy a close and trusting relationship with their patients as part of the care pact.

The recognition and protection of patients' rights reflects the evolution of ethical values and legal standards aimed at ensuring respect for human dignity in the medical field. It is therefore essential to reinforce doctors' training and awareness of these fundamental issues.

VI. References

1. World Health Organization. Constitution of the World Health Organization. 1946. Available at: https://apps.who.int/gb/bd/PDF/bd47/FR/constitution-fr.pdf.

2 United Nations General Assembly. Universal Declaration of Human Rights. 1948. Available at: https://www.un.org/fr/universal-declaration-human-rights/.

3. Adhikari S, Paudel K, Aro AR, Adhikari TB, Adhikari B, Mishra SR. Knowledge, attitude and practice of healthcare ethics among resident doctors and ward nurses from a resource poor setting, Nepal. BMC Med Ethics. dec 2016;17(1):68.

4. Constitution de la République Tunisienne 2022. Journal Officiel de la République Tunisienne n°91 du 18 aout 2022.

5 Law no. 91-63 of July 29, 1991 on health organization. Journal Officiel de la République Tunisienne n°51 du 02 aout 1991.

6. Tunisian Penal Code. Journal Officiel de la République Tunisienne . July 09, 1913.

7 The Tunisian Code of Ethics. Decree no. 93-1155 of May 17, 1993, on the code of medical ethics. JORT n° 40 of May 28 and June 1, 1993 page 764). 1993.

8. CHARTER OF FUNDAMENTAL RIGHTS OF THE EUROPEAN UNION. Official Journal of the European Union.2012/C 326/02. 2012. Available at: https://eur-lex.europa.eu/legal-content/FR/TXT/HTML/?uri=CELEX%3A12012P%2FTXT.

9 Decree No. 81-1634 of November 30, 1981, on the general internal regulations of hospitals. Journal Officiel de la République Tunisienne of December 4, 1981.

10 Law no. 92-71 of July 27, 1992, on communicable diseases.

11 International Covenant on Economic, Social and Cultural Rights. Available at: https://www.ohchr.org/fr/instruments-mechanisms/instruments/international-covenant-economic-social-and-culturalrights.

12. Tunisian Patient Charter. April 2010. Ministry of Health, Republic of Tunisia; pp. 1-4.

13. B. HOERNI. Medical ethics and deontology. 2nd edition Masson; 2000.

14 Ministry of Health decree of May 28, 2001 approving the specifications for private health establishments. Journal Officiel de la République Tunisienne n°46 du 08 juin 2001.

15. Handbook of Tunisian prison law. Ministry of Justice, Republic of Tunisia; 2019.

16. Meghalaya, Northeast India, et al. A study to Evaluate Knowledge of Handling Medico-Legal Cases among Interns in a Teaching Institution. Indian J Forensic Med Pathol. 2018;11(2):65-70.

17. Nath A, Ropmay A, Slong D, Patowary A, Rao A. A cross-sectional study on knowledge of registered medical practitioners, regarding management of medico-legal cases in Meghalaya. J Fam Med Prim Care. 2022;11(3):904.

18. Fadare J, Desalu O, Jemilohun A, Babatunde O. Knowledge of medical ethics among Nigerian medical doctors. Niger Med J. 2012;53(4):226.

19. G Venkat Rao, N Hari. Medico-legal knowledge assessment of interns and post graduate

students in a medical institution. IAIM 2016 310 105-110.

20. Mathew S, Samant N, Cooksey C, Ramm O. Knowledge, Attitudes, and Perceptions About Medicolegal Education: A Survey of OB/GYN Residents. Perm J. Dec 2020;24(5):19.217.

21 Aacharya RP, Shakya YL. Knowledge, attitude and practice of medical ethics among medical intern students in a Medical College in Kathmandu. Bangladesh J Bioeth. May 6, 2016;6(3):1-9.

22. Reddy PS, Abhinandana R. Awareness of Medicolegal Issues among Interns and Resident Doctors at a Tertiary Care Hospital in Kolar, Karnataka, India: A Cross-sectional Study. J Clin Diagn Res. 2023 ; Available at: https://www.jcdr.net//article_fulltext.asp?issn=0973-709x&year=2023&volume=17&issue=8&page=HC01&issn=0973-709x&id=18336

23 Law n° 91-22 of March 25, 1991, relating to the removal and transplantation of human organs. Journal Officiel de la République Tunisienne n°22 of March 29, 1991.

24. Aissaoui A. Evaluation of the knowledge of physicians practicing at the University Hospitals of Mahdia and Monastir in the field of patients' rights, 2018 [Dissertation]. FMM; 2018.

25 Gupta G, Singh AN, Bansal N, Wander GS. Knowledge about Informed Consent among Doctors of Various Specialities: A Pilot Survey. J Assoc Physicians India. oct 2018;66(10):57-62.

26. United Nations. Nelson Mandela Rules (Standard Minimum Rules for the Treatment of Prisoners). Available at: https://www.un.org/en/documents/decl_conv/conventions/treatment_prisoners.shtml.

27. Jeremić Stojković V, Cvjetković S, Matejić B. Physicians' Attitudes toward Adolescent Confidentiality Services: Scale Development and Validation. Slov J Public Health. June 1, 2020;59(2):99-107.

28. Law 2015-26 of August 07 relating to the fight against terrorism and the repression of money laundering. Journal Officiel de la République Tunisienne n°63 of August 07, 2015.

29 Decree-Law no. 2011-115 of November 2, 2011, on freedom of the press, printing and publishing. Journal Officiel de la République Tunisienne n° 84 du 04 novembre 2011 p. 2559-68.

30. Law n° 95-92 of November 9, 1995 relating to the publication of the child protection code. Journal Officiel de la République Tunisienne n°90 du 10 novembre 1995;(91):2063-2078. Available at: https://www.jurisitetunisie.com/tunisie/codes/cde/menu.html

31. Gabriela Kato Lettieri, Aline Hung Tai, Aline Rodrigues Hütter , André Luiz Torres Raszl , Mariana Moura 1,, Raquel Barbosa Cintra. Medical confidentiality in the digital era: an analysis of physician-patient relations. Rev Bioét Print Version ISSN 1983-8042 -Line Version ISSN 1983-8034.

32. Ketels B, Vander Beken T. MEDICAL CONFIDENTIALITY AND PARTNER NOTIFICATION IN CASES OF SEXUALLY TRANSMISSIBLE INFECTIONS IN BELGIUM. Med Law Rev. 1 Sep 2012;20(3):399-422.

33 United Nations Rules for the Treatment of Prisoners and Non-custodial Measures for Women Offenders (Bangkok Rules). Available at:

https://www.unodc.org/documents/justice-andprison-reform/BKKrules/UNODC_Bangkok_Rules_FRE_web.pdf.

34. Decree no. 2014-3657 of October 3, 2014, amending and supplementing decree no. 90-1401 of September 3, 1990, setting the terms and conditions for medical or scientific experimentation of medicines intended for human medicine.

35. González-Duarte A, Zambrano-González E, Medina-Franco H, Alberú-Gómez J, Durand-Carbajal M, Hinojosa CA, Aguilar-Salinas CA, Kaufer-Horwitz M. II. THE RESEARCH ETHICS INVOLVING VULNERABLE GROUPS. Rev Invest Clin. 2019;71(4):217-225. doi: 10.24875/RIC.19002812. PMID: 31448777.

36. Research Involving Pregnant Participants. Colorado: University of Colorado; 2022 Mar p. 1-6.

37. Pregnant women, scientific and ethical considerations for inclusion in clinical trials. 2018.

38. Gaddas M, Jedidi M, Ben Khelil M, Ben Saad H. Medical experimentation on prisoners (part 3):

the main milestones of the evolving ethical' texts and codes. Tunis Med. 2022;100(8-9):572-7.

39 Law n°2001-52 of May 14, 2001 relating to the organization of prisons. JORT n°40 of May 18, 2001.

VII.

VIII. Appendices

QUESTIONNAIRE

The question of medical and ethical health law is always topical, and is an important aspect of patient care.

The aim of this survey is to assess doctors' knowledge of medical and ethical health law. Please answer the following questionnaire.

*NB: you'll get the right answers as soon as you fill in the questionnaire.

Age :

Gender: M/F

Profession:

Médecin ☐

Résident en médecine ☐

AHU ☐

Spécialiste ☐

Pharmacien

Dentiste

☐

Have you attended a course or conference on a medical law topic?

NO YES If yes, which themes? ....

Have you attended a course or conference on the rights of persons deprived of their liberty?

NO YES

I. Patient rights and health ethics :

1. Consent to care :

a-Must be based on clear and fair information prior to any act of care

b-must be written

c-Est in most cases oral

d-Must be obtained by the legal guardian in the case of a minor or incapacitated adult e-Est obligatory on the part of the husband in the case of a voluntary interruption of pregnancy

Answer: a/c/d

2. Information :
   - a- A serious prognosis can be hidden from the patient
   - b- Terminal cancer can be delivered to a close family member
   - c- A transmissible disease such as AIDS can be hidden from the patient because of its psychological repercussions.
   - d- Mandatory even in emergencies

Answer: a/b

3. A patient admitted to your surgical department with simple vesicular lithiasis is requesting that she be operated on by the department head.
   - a. She does not have the right to choose her own doctor, regardless of the establishment (public or private).

b. You inform her that she will be operated on by the surgeon according to the organization of the department and the availability of surgeons.

Answer: b

4. A patient hospitalized in a public hospital wishes to continue his treatment in a polyclinic. He asks for his medical file:

   a. The care team is obliged to give him all his medical records.

   b. He is entitled to a copy of the discharge summary for continuity of care.

Answer: b

5. A 17-year-old girl, brought back to the ER by her parents following a spontaneous abortion, asks you not to inform her strict, conservative parents.

   a- You accept for its physical benevolence

   b- You inform them anyway

Answer: a

6. Caregivers must report to the authorities :

   a- Child abuse

   b- Violence against women

   c- Crime already committed

   d- Crime in the making

   Answer: a/b/d

7. A patient consults you and confesses that he has committed a criminal offence:

   a- You report the situation to the judicial authorities

   b- You maintain medical confidentiality and continue to provide the necessary medical care.

Answer: b

8. A boy went to the emergency room on suspicion of acute meningitis. On examination, the doctor found traces of physical violence of different ages. Urgent hospitalization is indicated, but the

father refuses and asks the medical team to write him a prescription.

a- You hospitalize the patient

b- Report the situation to the child protection delegate

c- You respect the wishes of the legal guardian

Answer: a/b

9. A patient is admitted to your department for therapy of an HIV infection . His wife requests information on her husband's state of health.

Are you going to inform him?

a- Yes

b- No

c- I don't know

Answer: b

10. Before starting any scientific drug research, the candidate's oral consent must be obtained, based

on clear information concerning the stages of the research and possible adverse effects:

a- Yes

b-No

c- I don't know

Answer: b

11. Pregnant women can be candidates for drug research:

a- Yes

b - No

c - I don't know

Answer: b

12. You receive a comatose, multi-targeted patient with end-stage breast cancer in the emergency department. Dr. A. refuses to intervene, as this is a hopeless case. Do you agree with him?

a- Yes

b-No

c- I don't know

Answer: b

13. Do you think that Dr. A. could be held liable in this case?

a- Yes

b- No

c- I don't know

Answer: a

14. A terminally ill neo patient asks you, as his physician, to help him die with dignity.

a- You accept

b- You refuse

c- You continue palliative treatment

Answer: b/c

II. Health rights of persons deprived of their liberty :

1. In the emergency department of a regional hospital, you receive a 22-year-old patient under arrest (handcuffed-accompanied by 2 police

officers) for head trauma following a fall from his own height.

The police tell you that he is in police custody on suspicion of involvement in acts of terrorism and that he is dangerous.

a. You ask for the patient's consent to examine him or her and provide the necessary care:

Oui ☐

Non ☐

Answer: yes

b. You ask the officers' permission to examine and treat a patient in police custody:

Oui ☐

Non ☐

Answer: no

2. A prisoner is hospitalized on your ward for treatment of an HIV infection. The police ask for information about his state of health.

Will you be informing them?

a- Yes

b- No

c- I don't know

Answer: b

3. A deathrow inmate tested positive for SARS Covid-19. He suddenly presented an alteration in his general condition with signs of respiratory struggle. The prison doctor refused to examine the patient, declaring "I categorically refuse to risk my life and catch the virus by trying to treat this murderer".

Do you agree with him?

a. Yes

b. No

c. I don't know

Answer: b

Do you think the doctor could be held criminally liable in this case?

a- Yes

b- No

c- I don't know

Answer: a

4. From an ethical point of view, prisoners can be candidates for clinical trials as part of medical research:

a- Yes

b- No

c- I don't know

Answer: b

Thank you for your cooperation

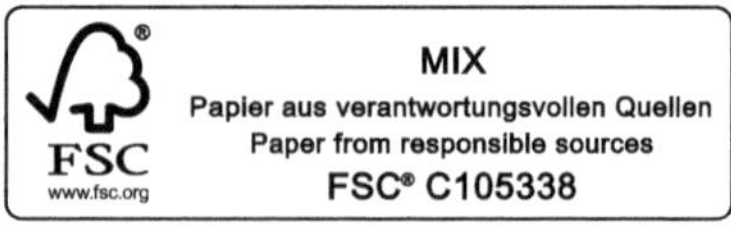

Printed by Books on Demand GmbH, Norderstedt / Germany